COPYRIGHT LAWRENCE ADKINS

Navigating Medicare: A Guide for Turning 65 Copyright 2024

Introduction copyright Lawrence Adkins All rights reserved. Printed in the United States of America. No part of this book may be used or reproduced in any manner whatsoever without written permission except in the case of brief quotations embodied in critical articles and reviews. For information address Golden Ray Publishing, FL. Books may be purchased for educational, business, or sales promotional use. For information on video and audio testimonials for reproduction contact: lisa@goldenraybooks.com

No part of this books publication may be reproduced, stored in a retrieval system, or transmitted in any form or by any means – electronic, mechanical, photocopying, recording or otherwise – without the written permission of the publisher.

Golden Ray Publishing

Cheyenne, Wyoming

www.goldenraybooks.com

> *This Book is Dedicated to everyone who turns 65 as you will become eligible for Medicare.*
>
> *This Book is your "How To" Guide for success I n pursuing a healthy life.*

INTRODUCTION

As you approach the milestone of turning 65, you are likely beginning to think about the next phase of your life, retirement. One of the most important decisions you will make during this time is related to your health insurance. Navigating the complexities of Medicare and understanding your options can feel overwhelming. It's a decision that can significantly impact your financial security and well-being for years to come, and it's one that should not be taken lightly. I've been in the financial planning industry since 1992, and over the years, I've had the privilege of helping thousands of individuals prepare for retirement. Throughout my career, I've held various roles, each offering me a deeper understanding of how crucial it is to build a strong financial foundation. And for many people, that foundation starts with making the right healthcare decisions.

As you move into retirement, health insurance is one of the most vital components of your overall financial plan. Without the right coverage, unexpected medical expenses can derail even the best laid plans. This book is written with you in mind—to help guide you through the often-complicated landscape of Medicare and healthcare options for seniors. There are many factors to consider when choosing the right plan for your needs, your health, medications, doctors, preferred hospitals, travel plans, and more. Each person's situation is unique, and there is no one-size-fits- all solution. That's why it's so important to educate yourself and make informed choices. My hope is that this book will provide you with the knowledge you need to make smart, well-informed decisions about your healthcare coverage as you enter retirement.

Whether you're considering traditional Medicare, Medicare Advantage, or Medi-gap supplement plans, understanding the pros

NAVIGATING

PURSUING A HEALTHY LIFE

MEDICARE

WHEN TURNING 65

A GUIDE

WRITTEN BY

LAWRENCE ADKINS

#1 BARNES AND NOBLE BESTSELLER

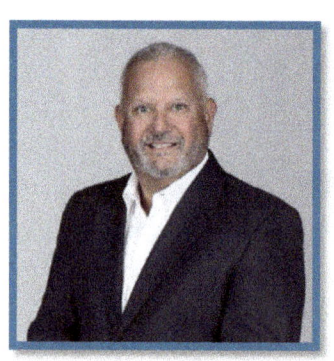

AUTHOR: LAWRENCE ADKINS

CEO ACBS INSURANCE SERVICES

ladkins@acbs-llc.com

http://www.acbsinsuranceservices.com/

"Our customers are at the heart of everything we do!"

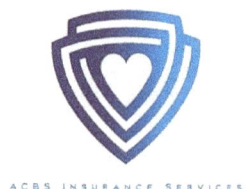

and cons of each option is essential for securing the coverage that works best for you and your lifestyle.

While this book will provide you with valuable information, I also strongly recommend that you seek guidance from an experienced professional, someone who can help you navigate the details and answer your questions along the way. Experienced agents, like those at ACBS Insurance, who collectively bring over 200 years of expertise to the table, can provide personalized advice and help you make the right Medicare choices for your unique circumstances. Your health insurance decisions in retirement are important, and I am confident that with the right resources, the right guidance, and a clear understanding of your options, you can make sure you can make an informed decision. At ACBS Insurance Services, we are a nationally recognized independent insurance agency dedicated to providing unbiased assistance and support to seniors and their families in selecting Medicare insurance plan options that best suit their needs and budget. Our mission is to bring peace of mind to those entering retirement by simplifying the complex and often confusing process of securing quality, affordable healthcare. We understand that the array of healthcare options available through Medicare can be overwhelming, and the importance of adhering to specific timeframes and enrollment windows to obtain crucial benefits cannot be overstated.

Seeing a gap in the insurance industry, ACBS Insurance Services was founded to offer a higher standard of service. As an independent agency representing a wide range of Medicare insurance plan options across the United States, we provide impartial guidance to help our clients choose the most appropriate coverage tailored to their unique situations. Through education, professional qualifications, and market analysis, we ensure our clients are well-informed and confident in their healthcare decisions. Our independence means our loyalty lies solely with our clients, not any insurance company. Our goal is to empower individuals with the knowledge they need to make the best healthcare choices. We serve as a dedicated point of contact and advocate, guiding our clients through every step of the enrollment process and continually reassessing their coverage to adapt to changing needs, ensuring they always have the best possible insurance fit. Thank you for allowing me to share this information with you, and I wish you success and peace of mind as you move into this exciting new chapter of your life 65 and over.

Lawrence Adkins
CEO / ACBS Insurance Services

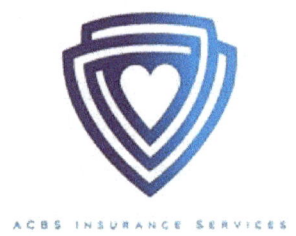

Why This Guide Matters:

Turning 65 is not just a numerical milestone; it's a pivotal moment in your life that signifies many changes, especially regarding your healthcare coverage. For many, the complexity of Medicare can be overwhelming. The decisions you make now will directly affect your healthcare coverage for the rest of your life, making it essential to understand all the available options and how they work together.

Choosing the right Medicare plan is not just about meeting immediate healthcare needs but also about anticipating future needs. This guide is designed to help you. By the end of this guide, you will have the confidence to select the plan that is best for you.

Turning 65: What It Means for Health Insurance:

When you turn 65, you will become eligible for Medicare. However, you won't necessarily be enrolled right away unless you're already receiving Social Security benefits. If you are still employed, you may also be able to delay enrolling in Medicare without facing penalties. Understanding when to enroll and which parts of Medicare to choose can be confusing, but it's critical to get it right. Medicare provides coverage for hospital care, medical services, and prescription drugs, but it is not a one-size-fits-all solution.

There are various parts to consider, and each offers different levels of coverage. In this book, we will break down each part of Medicare in detail, so you can make the most informed decision.

CONTENTS

1. UNDERSTANDING MEDICARE BASICS   1
2. ENROLLING IN MEDICARE   5
3. MEDICARE PART A & PART B   8
4. SUPPLEMENTAL COVERAGE OPTIONS   13
5. PRESCRIPTION DRUG COVERAGE (PART D)   19
6. FINANCIAL CONSIDERATIONS IN MEDICARE   24
7. USING MEDICARE WISELY   28
8. FREQUENTLY ASKED QUESTIONS   31
9. RESOURCES FOR MEDICARE ASSISTANCE   33

ABOUT THE AUTHOR   48

How to Use This Book: The 9 Steps for Success

This guide is structured to provide step-by-step advice on understanding and navigating Medicare, with each chapter focusing on a specific aspect of the program.

Chapter 1: Understanding Medicare Basics.

This chapter explains the basics of Medicare, how it works, and the different parts of the program.

Chapter 2: Enrolling in Medicare: This chapter walks you through the enrollment process, from understanding when to enroll to how to sign up for coverage.

Chapter 3: Medicare Part A And Part B.

This chapter gives you an in-depth look at Medicare Parts A and B, the core components of Original Medicare.

Chapter 4: Supplemental Coverage Options explore your supplemental coverage options, including Medigap and Medicare Advantage, to ensure you get the coverage you need.

Chapter 5: Prescription Drug Coverage (Part D) discusses prescription drug coverage (Part D), so you can understand how to manage your medications and avoid unnecessary costs.

Chapter 6: Chapter 6: Financial Considerations in Medicare covers the financial aspects of Medicare, including out-of-pocket costs, budgeting, and available financial assistance programs.

Chapter 7: Using Medicare Wisely offers practical advice on using Medicare effectively, such as finding providers, utilizing preventive care, and handling billing disputes.

Chapter 8: Frequently Asked Questions address frequently asked questions, common mistakes to avoid, and tips for making the most of your Medicare benefits.

Chapter 9: Resources for Medicare Assistance provides a list of valuable resources, including websites, phone numbers, and organizations that can help you manage your Medicare coverage.

1
UNDERSTANDING MEDICARE BASICS

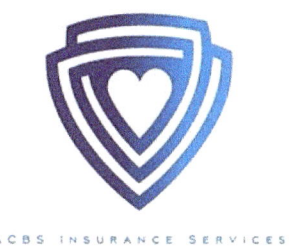

ACBS INSURANCE SERVICES

What is Medicare?

Medicare is a federal health insurance program that provides coverage for individuals aged 65 and older, as well as younger people with certain disabilities or chronic conditions. It is designed to help reduce the financial burden of healthcare in retirement, covering a range of services from hospital stays, outpatient care, medical equipment, and prescription drugs. **Medicare is divided into four main parts: Part A, Part B, Part C, and Part D. Each part covers different types of care and services.**

Medicare Part A (Hospital Insurance): This part of Medicare covers hospital stays, skilled nursing facility care, hospice care, and some home health care. Most people qualify for premium-free Part A if they or their spouse paid Medicare taxes while working.

Medicare Part B (Medical Insurance): Part B covers outpatient services, such as doctor visits, outpatient hospital services, certain preventive services, and medical supplies. Part B requires a monthly premium that varies depending on your income.

Medicare Part C (Medicare Advantage): Medicare Advantage is an alternative to Original Medicare (Parts A and B). These plans are offered by private insurers and often include additional benefits like prescription drug coverage (Part D), vision, dental, and wellness programs.

Medicare Part D (Prescription Drug Coverage, PDP): Part D helps cover the cost of prescription drugs. Part D plans are offered by private insurance companies and are optional, though you may incur penalties if you don't sign up when you're first eligible.

How Medicare Works

Medicare offers two primary options for receiving benefits: Original Medicare and Medicare Advantage. Understanding the differences between the two is crucial in deciding which one will meet your needs. **Original Medicare**: This includes Part A and Part B. With original Medicare, you can go to any doctor or hospital that accepts Medicare, and you generally don't need referrals for specialist visits. However, Original Medicare doesn't cover everything. It doesn't cover prescription drugs, vision, dental care, or hearing aids, which is why many people also enroll in a value-added benefits plan, either a Medigap policy or a Part D plan.

Medicare Advantage: Medicare Advantage plans (Part C) are offered by private insurance companies and cover everything Original Medicare covers, and often more. These plans usually include prescription drug coverage (Part D), and some plans may offer additional services such as vision, dental, and hearing coverage. However, they typically have network restrictions and require you to use doctors and hospitals within the plan's network.

Key Medicare Terms

It's important to familiarize yourself with key Medicare terminology to avoid confusion later. Some of the most important terms include:

Premium: The monthly payment you make to Medicare or a private insurer for coverage. For example, you pay a premium for Part B (medical insurance) and may also pay for Part D

(prescription drug coverage).

Deductible: The amount you may pay for covered health care services before your Medicare plan begins to pay.

Copayments and Coinsurance: A copayment is a fixed amount you pay for a service, while coinsurance is the percentage of the cost you must pay for a service. For example, after meeting your deductible, you might pay 20% of the cost for outpatient services under Part B, which is your coinsurance.

Out-of-Pocket Maximum: Medicare Advantage plans offer an out-of-pocket maximum, which caps the amount you'll have to pay for covered services in a year. This can be particularly valuable in controlling healthcare expenses, as Original Medicare does not have an out-of-pocket maximum.

2
ENROLLING IN MEDICARE

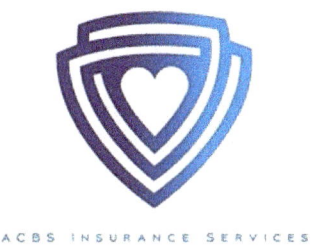

Who Needs to Enroll?

When you turn 65, you may be automatically enrolled in Medicare if you are already receiving Social Security or Railroad Retirement benefits. However, if you are not receiving these benefits, you will need to manually enroll in Medicare.

If you are still working and have health insurance through your employer, you may be able to delay enrollment in Part B without facing a penalty.

However, once you stop working or lose your employer coverage, you'll need to enroll within 8 months to avoid penalties.

When to Enroll

There are specific periods during which you can enroll in Medicare:

Initial Enrollment Period (IEP): This is a 7-month period that starts 3 months before your 65th birthday, includes the month of your birthday, and ends 3 months after your birthday. If you enroll during this period, you can start your coverage on the first day of the month when you turn 65.

Special Enrollment Period (SEP): If you are covered under an employer's health insurance plan, you may qualify for a Special Enrollment Period when you retire or lose that coverage. You may not face a late enrollment penalty if you enroll during this period.

General Enrollment Period: If you miss your Initial Enrollment Period, you can sign up during the General Enrollment Period (from January 1 to March 31 each year). However, if you enroll during this period, your coverage won't begin until July 1, and you may face late enrollment penalties.

Late Enrollment Penalties: If you fail to enroll in Part B or Part D when you're first eligible, you could face penalties. The penalty for Part B is 10% for each year you delay enrollment, and the penalty for Part D is 1% of the national average premium for each month you delay.

How to Enroll

Enrolling in Medicare is a straightforward process. You can apply online through the Social Security Administration's website, by phone, or in person at a local Social Security office.

Online: Visit the Social Security website (www.ssa.gov) to complete your application.

By Phone: Call Social Security at 1-800-772-1213 to enroll over the phone.

In Person: You can also visit a Social Security office to apply in person. When you apply, you'll need to provide basic information, such as your date of birth, Social Security number, and proof of U.S. citizenship or legal residency.

Glossary of Terms

Premium: The amount you pay each month for your Medicare coverage. Deductible: The amount you pay for healthcare services before Medicare begins to pay.

Coinsurance: The percentage of costs you pay after meeting your deductible.

Copayment: A fixed amount you pay for a covered healthcare service. Formulary: A list of medications covered by a Medicare drug plan.

3

MEDICARE PART A & PART B

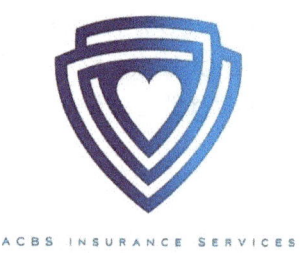

Medicare Part A (Hospital Insurance)

Medicare Part A is one of the cornerstones of the Medicare program. It helps pay for hospital stays, skilled nursing facility care, hospice care, and certain home health services. In most cases, if you or your spouse paid Medicare taxes while working, you won't have to pay a premium for

Part A—this is often called premium-free Part A. However, even if you qualify for premium- free Part A, you may still have to pay for certain services.

What's Covered by Part A?

Inpatient hospital care: This includes room and board, general nursing care, meals, and most of your hospital services while you're an inpatient. Medicare Part A covers stays in a general hospital, a psychiatric hospital, or a critical access hospital. Skilled nursing facility care: If you need skilled care after a hospital stay, Part A covers up to 100 days of skilled nursing care in a facility (for rehabilitation or recovery). However, the first 20 days are fully covered, and from days 21 to 100, there's a daily coinsurance.

Hospice care: Part A covers hospice services for terminally ill patients who are expected to live six months or less. Hospice care includes pain relief, palliative care, and support for the patient's family.

Home health care: If you are homebound and need skilled services like physical therapy for nursing care, Part A may cover the costs, though certain conditions apply. Costs of Part A For most people, Part A comes without a premium. However, if you didn't work or pay Medicare taxes for at least 40 quarters (10 years), you may have to pay a premium for Part A. Additionally, there are other costs associated with Part A that you'll need to understand:

Deductible: For each benefit period (which is a period during which you are receiving care), you must pay the Part A deductible. For 2026, Part A deductible is $1,804 per benefit period.

Coinsurance: After the deductible, you may need to pay coinsurance. For example, for hospital stays of more than 60 days, you'll pay a daily coinsurance cost, which increases the longer your stay.

Limitations of Part A

While Part A covers a lot of inpatient care, it doesn't cover everything. For instance, it doesn't pay for private-duty nurses, personal care items like toiletries, or most dental, vision, and hearing services. Therefore, many people also consider additional coverage to fill these gaps.

Medicare Part B (Medical Insurance)

Medicare Part B is the part of Medicare that covers outpatient care and services that are medically necessary, such as doctor visits, outpatient surgeries, diagnostic tests, and some preventive care. Unlike Part A, Part B comes with a monthly premium that is based on your income.

What's Covered by Part B?

Doctor services: Medicare Part B covers physician visits, both in the office and when you're hospitalized (if the service is medically necessary). It also covers some specialists and specialists, visits.

Outpatient hospital services: Part B covers outpatient services you receive at a hospital, such as outpatient surgeries or emergency room visits.

Preventive services: Medicare covers a range of preventive services, including screenings for cancer (e.g., mammograms), flu shots, and vaccinations.

Medical equipment: Part B covers medically necessary durable medical equipment (DME) such as wheelchairs, walkers, oxygen equipment, and certain other devices.

Mental health services: Medicare covers outpatient mental health services, such as counseling and therapy, provided by psychiatrists, clinical psychologists, and clinical social workers.

Home health care: While Part A covers skilled nursing care at home, Part B can help pay for medically necessary services not covered by Part A, such as physical therapy or durable medical equipment.

Costs of Part B

Premiums: Most people pay a standard premium for Part B, which is deducted from your Social Security check. For 2026, the standard Part B premium is $206.50 per month. However, if you have a higher income, you may pay an Income-Related Monthly Adjustment Amount (IRMAA), which increases your premium.

Deductible: In addition to the monthly premium, you will pay an annual deductible of $288 for Part B services. After you meet your deductible, you pay 20% of the Medicare- approved amount for most doctor visits, outpatient therapy, and durable medical equipment.

Coinsurance: After meeting your deductible, you'll pay 20% of the Medicare-approved amount for most services. However, this can vary depending on the specific service you need.

Limitations of Part B

While Part B covers a broad range of outpatient services, it doesn't cover everything. For instance, it doesn't cover prescription drugs (unless they are administered in a clinical setting), dental care, routine vision exams, or hearing aids. To cover these gaps, you may need to consider a Medicare Advantage plan or a Medigap policy.

Deciding on Part A and Part B

Most people will be automatically enrolled in Part A if they receive Social Security Benefits. However, enrolling in Part B is a personal choice. Some people who are still working and have employer-sponsored health insurance may choose to delay Part B enrollment without facing a penalty. However, if you are not covered by an employer's plan or are retired, enrolling in both Parts A and B is generally advisable.

If you are on a tight budget, you may want to consider the financial aspects of both parties. For example, if you don't need much medical care, you may find that paying the monthly Part B premium is not worthwhile, but if you expect to need more medical care, having both Part A and Part B can give you much-needed coverage for a broader range of services.

4

SUPPLEMENTAL COVERAGE OPTIONS

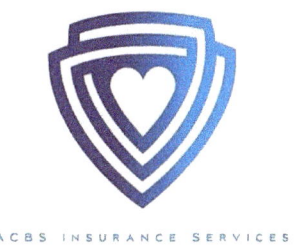

Medigap (Medicare Supplement Insurance)

Medigap is private health insurance that can be added to Original Medicare (Parts A and B) to help cover the gaps left by Medicare, such as deductibles, coinsurance, and copayments. Medigap policies are sold by private insurance companies and are standardized, meaning that the benefits are the same no matter which insurer you buy from. However, the cost of Medigap policies can vary from insurer to insurer.

What Medigap Covers

Medigap plans cover some or all the out-of-pocket costs that Original Medicare doesn't cover, including Coinsurance: After you meet your deductible, Medigap can cover the 20% coinsurance that you would otherwise be responsible for.

Copayments: Some plans can help with copayments for services like doctor visits, hospital stays, and emergency care.

Deductibles: Medigap can cover your Part A deductible, as well as your Part B deductible in some plans.

Foreign Travel Emergency Coverage: Some Medigap plans also offer emergency medical coverage when you travel outside the U.S.

Medigap Plans: A Through N

Medigap policies are standardized into plans labeled A through N. Each plan offers a different level of coverage, so you can choose a plan based on how much coverage you need and how much you're willing to pay in premiums.

For example: Plan F (the most comprehensive option) covers the full Part A deductible, Part B deductible, and all coinsurance, as well as coverage for foreign travel emergencies.

Plan G is another popular plan, covering everything except the Part B deductible.

Plan N offers less comprehensive coverage and typically has lower premiums but requires more out-of-pocket costs for office visits and some hospital services.

Costs of Medigap

The cost of a Medigap policy depends on several factors, including where you live, your age, gender, tobacco use, and the plan you choose. Although Medigap helps cover your Medicare gaps, you'll need to pay a monthly premium on top of your Part B premium.

How to Choose a Medigap Plan

When deciding whether to purchase a Medigap plan, it's important to consider your health needs, financial situation, and preferred level of coverage. If you anticipate frequent doctor visits or hospital stays, Medigap can be a valuable way to help manage your healthcare costs. However, if you're relatively healthy and want to save on premiums, a lower-level Medigap plan may be a good fit.

Medicare Advantage (Part C)

Medicare Advantage plans (Part C) are another way to receive your Medicare benefits. These plans are offered by private insurance companies and combine coverage from both Medicare

Parts A and B and often include prescription drug coverage (Part D).

What Medicare Advantage Covers

Hospital Care (Part A): Includes inpatient care, skilled nursing care, hospice care, and home health services. Medical Services (Part B): Includes outpatient care, doctor visits, preventive services, and some medical equipment.

Prescription Drugs (Part D): Most Medicare Advantage plans include Part D coverage, which helps pay for prescription medications.

Additional Benefits of Medicare Advantage

Many Medicare Advantage plans also offer extra benefits that are not covered by Original Medicare, such as:

Dental: Coverage for routine dental care, like cleanings, exams, and X-rays.

Vision: Coverage for eye exams, glasses, or contact lenses. Hearing: Coverage for hearing exams and hearing aids.

Fitness: Many plans include access to fitness programs or gyms.

These added benefits can be a significant draw for those who need or want more comprehensive coverage.

Costs of Medicare Advantage

Unlike Original Medicare, Medicare Advantage plans have a premium (in addition to your Part B premium) that varies by plan. Some plans offer low or $0 premiums, but you will still be responsible for copays, deductibles, and coinsurance for services. Additionally, these plans usually have an annual out-of-pocket maximum, which can protect you from excessive medical costs.

Medicare Advantage: Pros and Cons

Pros:

- All-in-one coverage (Part A, B, D, and extra benefits).
- Often includes prescription drug coverage.
- May offer additional services like dental and vision.
- Low or $0 premium plans.

Cons:

- Limited to a specific network of doctors and hospitals.
- You may need referrals to see specialists.
- Higher out-of-pocket costs for some services.

If you are comfortable with managed care (network restrictions, referrals, and copays), Medicare Advantage can be a good option. However, if you prefer more flexibility in choosing providers, Original Medicare with Medigap might be a better fit.

Chapter Summary:

Medicare Parts A and B form the backbone of the Medicare program, but they do have gaps in coverage. Medigap and Medicare Advantage plans are two options for filling these gaps, and each comes with its pros and cons. When deciding between Original Medicare with Medigap or a Medicare Advantage plan, it's crucial to consider your health, financial situation, and preferences for flexibility and additional benefits. Absolutely! Let's continue expanding the remaining chapters to ensure that each chapter provides in-depth details, helpful tips, and practical advice to ensure you get the most out of your Medicare experience.

5
PRESCRIPTION DRUG COVERAGE (PART D)

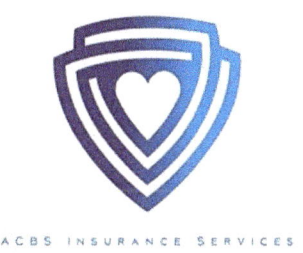

Chapter 5: Understanding Medicare Part D in 2026 – Your Guide to Prescription Drug Coverage

Medicare can feel like alphabet soup—Part A, Part B, Part C... and then there's Part D. If you take any prescription medications, Medicare Part D is the piece of the puzzle you need to understand. In this chapter, we'll walk you through how Medicare Part D works in 2026, in plain language—no jargon, no confusion.

What Is Medicare Part D?

Medicare Part D is insurance for prescription drugs. It helps cover the cost of the medications your doctor prescribes, anything from cholesterol pills to insulin, blood pressure medications to inhalers.

Part D is optional, but if you don't sign up when you're first eligible and try to join later, you might have to pay a late enrollment penalty every month for as long as you have coverage. So, even if you don't take many medications now, it's smart to consider enrolling when you become eligible.

Who Offers Part D Plans?

Here's something important: Medicare itself doesn't run Part D plans. Instead, it approves private insurance companies to offer these plans. So, when you shop for a Part D plan, you're choosing from different companies—like Aetna, Humana, UnitedHealthcare, and others—each with its own list of covered drugs and costs. That means your neighbor's plan might be different from yours— and that's okay. You want a plan that fits your medications and your budget.

In 2026, Medicare Part D changed for the better. Let's break it down step by step:

1. Monthly Premium

You pay a monthly fee to have the plan. In 2026, average premiums are around $30–$60 per month, but this varies by plan and where you live.

2. Annual Deductible

Some plans have a deductible—this is the amount you pay out-of-pocket before the plan begins helping. In 2026, the maximum deductible is $615. Some plans will waive this or lower it for certain drug tiers.

3. Copays and Coinsurance

After your deductible (if any), you start paying a copay (a fixed amount like $10 or $25) or coinsurance (a percentage, like 25%) when you fill prescriptions. This varies by the type of drug.

Plans group drugs into tiers—like a ladder:

- Tier 1: Low-cost generics (lowest copay)
- Tier 2: Preferred brand-name drugs
- Tier 3: Non-preferred brand drugs (higher copay)
- Tier 4: Specialty drugs (most expensive)

The Big Change in 2026: No More "Donut Hole"

Until recently, Medicare Part D had a confusing middle stage called the coverage gap or "donut hole," where you had to pay more for your prescriptions after reaching a certain limit.

As of 2025, that gap is gone. There's now a $2,100 annual out of pocket cap on what you'll pay for covered prescription drugs. That means:

- Once you spend $2,100 out of your own pocket (including deductible, copays, and coinsurance), you pay nothing for the rest of the year.

- This cap resets each January.

This is huge. It gives peace of mind to people who need expensive medications, especially those with chronic conditions like cancer, diabetes, or rheumatoid arthritis.

Extra Help for Low Incomes

If you have limited income and resources, you might qualify for a program called Extra Help, which can dramatically reduce your premiums, deductibles, and drug costs.

In 2026, more people qualify because the income limits have been raised. If you think you might be eligible, it's worth applying. A licensed agent or Medicare counselor can help you do it.

How to Pick the Right Plan

Here are 4 tips for choosing your Part D plan:

1. Make a list of your current medications—include the name, dosage, and how often you take them.

2. Use Medicare's Plan Finder tool at Medicare.gov to compare plans based on your medications and pharmacy.

3. Check the plan's drug formulary (list of covered drugs) to make sure your meds are included.

4. Ask a licensed agent for help. They can explain fine print and find a plan that fits your needs at no cost to you.

Real Life Example

Let's say Susan turns 65 in July and signs up for a Part D plan that costs $35/month. She takes a generic blood pressure pill and a brand-name cholesterol drug.

- Her deductible is $200. She hit that by March.
- After that, she pays $10/month for her generic and $40/month for the brand-name.
- By November, she's hit the $2,100 cap. In December, her medications cost nothing out of pocket.

Simple. Predictable. No surprises.

Final Thoughts

Part D can seem complicated, but in 2026, it's become a lot more manageable. With the new $2,100 cap, more generous financial assistance, and competitive private plan options, Medicare Part D is one of the most valuable pieces of your healthcare safety net. Understanding it is the first step. Choosing wisely is the next. And if you ever need help, don't go it alone—use a trusted advisor who specializes in Medicare. You'll be glad you did.

FINANCIAL CONSIDERATIONS IN MEDICARE

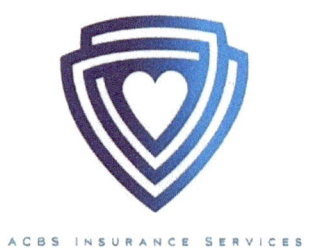

Understanding Costs in Medicare:

While Medicare provides significant help in covering healthcare expenses, it's important to remember that it doesn't cover everything. Understanding the costs associated with Medicare will help you manage your healthcare budget and avoid surprising expenses.

Premiums

A premium is a monthly fee you pay to maintain your Medicare coverage. You will pay a premium for Part B (medical insurance), and if you choose Medicare Advantage or Part D, you'll pay an additional premium for those plans. The cost of premiums varies depending on the plan, but the standard Part B premium for 2026 is $206.50 per month. If you have a higher income, you'll pay more due to an Income-Related Monthly Adjustment Amount (IRMAA).

Deductibles and Coinsurance

Medicare also requires you to pay deductibles and coinsurance for certain services. For example, in 2026, the Part A deductible is $1,804 per benefit period, and the Part B deductible is $288 annually.

Coinsurance is the percentage of the cost you pay after meeting your deductible. For example, for hospital stays under Part A, you will pay coinsurance after day 60 of your stay. Copayments are a fixed cost you pay for certain services, such as a doctor's visit.

Out-of-Pocket Maximums

If you choose a Medicare Advantage plan, one benefit is the out-of-pocket maximum. Once you've reached this limit, your plan covers 100% of the costs for covered services. Original Medicare does not have an out-of-pocket maximum, which can leave you exposed to high healthcare costs if you need frequent care.

Medicare Savings Programs

Medicare Savings Programs (MSPs) are designed to help lower income Medicare beneficiaries pay for certain out-of-pocket costs, including premiums, deductibles, and coinsurance. These programs are administered by state Medicaid programs, and eligibility is based on your income and assets.

Qualified Medicare Beneficiary (QMB):

This program helps with Part A and Part B premiums, deductibles, coinsurance, and copayments.

Specified Low-Income Medicare Beneficiary (SLMB): This program helps pay for Part B premiums.

Qualified Individual (QI): This program helps pay for Part B premiums for people who have slightly higher incomes than those eligible for SLMB. Medicaid and Dual Eligibility Some people with limited income and resources may also qualify for Medicaid. Medicaid is a state and federal program that provides additional assistance for healthcare costs. People who qualify for both Medicare and Medicaid are referred to as dual eligibles. These individuals often receive comprehensive coverage with minimal out-of-pocket costs.

Extra Help Program for Prescription Drug Costs

The Extra Help program helps people with limited income and resources pay for their Part D prescription drug costs. This program can assist with paying your Part D premium, deductible, coinsurance, and copayments. If you qualify, you will be automatically enrolled in Extra Help, and you may pay lower premiums and out-of-pocket costs for prescriptions.

7
USING MEDICARE WISELY

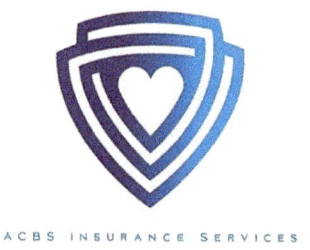

Navigating Providers and Services

Medicare gives you a lot of flexibility when choosing providers and services, but there are some rules and restrictions you need to be aware of, depending on whether you have Original Medicare or Medicare Advantage. Original Medicare with Original Medicare (Parts A and B), you can generally see any doctor or healthcare provider who accepts Medicare. This flexibility is one of the biggest advantages of Original Medicare, as you don't have to worry about network restrictions. However, there are some important things to remember:

No referrals: You don't need a referral to see a specialist.

Medicare assignment: Most providers accept Medicare assignments, which means they agree to the Medicare-approved amount for services. However, some may charge you more than the Medicare approved amount, which you'll need to pay out-of-pocket.

Medicare Advantage

Medicare Advantage plans often have network restrictions. For instance, some plans may require you to get care from doctors or hospitals within the plan's network, and you may need a referral to see a specialist. Make sure to check the network before enrolling in a plan to ensure it includes your preferred providers.

Preventive Services

Medicare provides many preventive services at no cost to help keep you healthy. These services are designed to detect health problems early when they are easier and less expensive to treat.

Examples of covered preventive services include:

Flu shots and other immunizations.

Cancer screenings such as mammograms, colonoscopies, and prostate exams.

Wellness visits to create a plan for managing your health. Diabetes and heart disease screenings.

Using preventive services is an important way to stay healthy and potentially avoid costly medical treatments down the road.

Medicare Timeline and Enrollment Periods

1. Initial Enrollment Period (IEP): This is the 7-month period when you first become eligible for Medicare. It starts 3 months before your 65th birthday month and ends 3 months after.

2. Annual Open Enrollment Period (AEP): October 15 to December 7. During this period, you can change your Medicare Advantage or Part D plans.

3. Special Enrollment Period (SEP): You may qualify for a SEP if you experience life events, like moving or losing employer coverage.

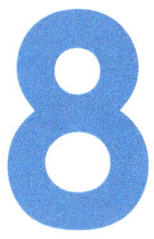

FREQUENTLY ASKED QUESTIONS

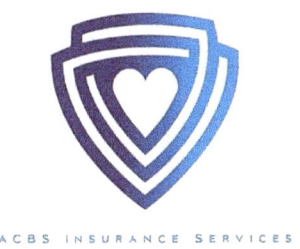

FAQs about Medicare:

1. What's the difference between Original Medicare and Medicare Advantage?

    o   Original Medicare includes Parts A and B, which you can use at any doctor or hospital that accepts Medicare. Medicare Advantage (Part C) is an all-in-one plan that often includes extra benefits and drug coverage, but it usually comes with a network of providers.

2. When should I enroll in Medicare?

    o   You should enroll in Medicare three months before your 65th birthday. If you're still working and have employer health insurance, you may be able to delay enrollment without penalties.

3. Do I need a supplemental plan if I have Medicare Advantage?

    o   No, if you have a Medicare Advantage, you don't need a Medigap policy. Medicare Advantage plans are designed to cover the gaps in Medicare, including coinsurance and deductibles.

4. What do I do if my Medicare claim is denied?

    o   If Medicare denies a claim, you can file an appeal. Start by reviewing the Explanation of Benefits (EOB) and the denial letter. You can appeal by following the instructions on the letter or by contacting Medicare directly.

RESOURCES FOR MEDICARE ASSISTANCE

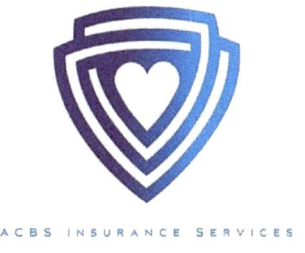

Where to Find Help

Navigating Medicare can be complicated, but fortunately, there are several resources available to help you make informed decisions about your coverage. Whether you need help understanding your options, comparing plans, or resolving billing issues, there are trusted sources to guide you.

State Health Insurance Assistance Programs (SHIP)

One of the best resources available to people with Medicare is the State Health Insurance Assistance Program (SHIP). SHIP is a nationwide network of free, unbiased counseling services that help Medicare beneficiaries understand their rights and options. These programs are run by each state, and counselors are trained to provide personalized guidance on a variety of Medicare-related topics. Whether you need help with enrollment, comparing plans, understanding coverage, or dealing with Medicare denials, SHIP counselors are there to assist you at no cost.

To find your state's SHIP, visit the SHIP National Technical Assistance Center website (www.shiptacenter.org) or call

1800-MEDICARE for more information.

Medicare's Helpline:

Medicare provides a dedicated helpline that you can call for assistance. Whether you have questions about enrolling in Medicare, want to understand your benefits, or need help with an issue related to your coverage, the Medicare helpline offers support.

The Medicare helpline is available at 1-800-MEDICARE (1-800633-4227). TTY users should call 1-877-486-2048. Representatives are available 24 hours a day, 7 days a week. Medicare.gov Website

The official Medicare.gov website is one of the most useful resources for finding information about your Medicare coverage. It offers comprehensive tools and resources, including Plan Finder Tool: Use this tool to compare Medicare Advantage plans, Part D prescription drug plans, and Medigap policies based on your specific needs and location.

Enrollment Resources: Step-by-step instructions on how to enroll in Medicare and related programs.

Coverage Information: Detailed descriptions of the different types of coverage available under Medicare, including Parts A, B, C, and D. Forms and Publications: Access the most up-to-date publications on Medicare policies, plan choices, and rights.

Local Agencies and Nonprofits

In addition to SHIP and the Medicare helpline, many local agencies and nonprofit organizations aid with Medicare related issues. These organizations may be particularly helpful for individuals with limited income who need assistance with enrollment, understanding costs, and applying for financial assistance programs.

Local Area Agencies on Aging (AAA) and Medicare Rights Centers can offer valuable resources for beneficiaries who need help understanding their options and accessing healthcare.

Family and Caregiver Support

If you have family members or caregivers who assist with managing your healthcare, they can be invaluable resources in helping you navigate Medicare. Be sure to include them in any decision-making about your coverage. This support system can help ensure that you understand the costs, coverage, and any deadlines associated with your Medicare choices.

Helpful Tools and Websites

There are several online tools and websites that can make navigating Medicare much easier. Here are some points listed for you to consider below:

Medicare Plan Finder

The Medicare Plan Finder tool on Medicare.gov is one of the most helpful resources available for comparing Medicare Advantage plans, Part D plans, and Medigap policies. You can enter your medications, preferred pharmacies, and health providers to get a list of plans available in your area, along with detailed costs and coverage information. This tool allows you to compare plans based on:

Premiums (monthly costs)

Out-of-pocket costs (deductibles, copayments, coinsurance) coverage details (specific medications, doctors, and hospitals covered) Medicare Savings Programs Eligibility Check

To help low-income individuals understand if they are eligible for additional financial assistance, the Medicare Savings Programs (MSPs) eligibility tool on the Medicare.gov website is a great resource. You can check if you qualify for programs that help pay for Medicare premiums, deductibles, and other out-of-pocket costs.

Online Prescription Drug Cost Calculators

Several websites allow you to calculate the cost of medications under various Part D plans and compare your options. This is particularly helpful for those on multiple medications, as the cost prescriptions can vary significantly across different plans.

Medicare's Online Cost Estimator

Medicare also offers an online cost estimator tool that allows you to get an idea of what your out-of-pocket costs may be for hospital visits, doctor's appointments, and other services based on your chosen plan. This tool considers the plan's premiums, deductibles, copayments, and coinsurance to help you budget for your healthcare needs.

Sample Questions to Ask Insurance Providers

What is the monthly premium for this plan? Are my doctors included in the plan's network? Does the plan cover my prescriptions?

What is the annual deductible for this plan? How much will I pay for a specialist visit?

Checklist for New Enrollees

Sign up for Medicare 3 months before turning 65.

Decide if you need Part A and Part B or if you want a Medicare Advantage plan. Review your current health needs and decide if you need additional coverage like Medigap or Part D.

Use the Medicare Plan Finder tool to compare plans. Contact SHIP for personalized guidance.

Staying Updated

Medicare is not a static program; it changes every year. Costs, coverage options, and rules may be updated annually, so it is crucial to stay informed to avoid unnecessary surprises.

Annual Open Enrollment Period (AEP)

Every year, from October 15 to December 7, Medicare beneficiaries can review and adjust their coverage during the Annual Open Enrollment Period (AEP). During this period, you can:

Change from Original Medicare to Medicare Advantage (or vice versa). Switch between Medicare Advantage plans.

Change your Part D prescription drug plan that best suits you.

Review any changes to your current plan, including premiums, deductibles, and covered services. Even if you're satisfied with your current plan, it's a good idea to review it each year. Plan benefits, premiums, and networks can change, and you might find a better option during the open enrollment period.

Medicare You Handbook

Each year, Medicare sends out the Medicare book; Your handbook to benefits. This publication provides an overview of Medicare's benefits, costs, and changes for the upcoming year. It's a great resource for keeping up with new developments in Medicare, and it's available online at the Medicare.gov website. To ensure you don't miss important updates, make sure your contact information is up to date with Medicare. You can sign up to receive updates via email or keep an eye on the mail for your annual notices. Medicare can be complex, but by taking advantage of available resources, staying informed, and using tools like the Medicare Plan Finder, you can make the best choices for your healthcare needs. Don't hesitate to reach out for help when you need it. Resources like SHIP, the Medicare helpline, and online tools can guide you through the process and help you find the coverage that fits your health, budget, and preferences.

Remember, it is important to review your Medicare coverage regularly. Changes to your health needs, prescription medications, and available plans may require adjustments to your coverage. With the right support and information, you can navigate the Medicare system with confidence.

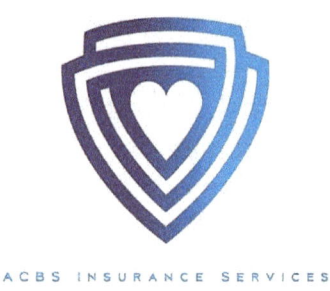

ACBS INSURANCE SERVICES

Navigating Medicare can feel overwhelming, but with the right information and resources, you can make informed decisions about your coverage. Take your time to review your options, seek assistance when needed, and stay on top of important dates like enrollment periods. By staying informed and proactive, you can ensure that you're getting the most out of your Medicare benefits and that your healthcare needs are well-managed in your later years.

REACH OUT FOR MORE INFORMATION:

LAWRENCE ADKINS ladkins@acbs-llc.com

http://www.acbsinsuranceservices.com/

"Our customers are at the heart of everything we do!"

ACBS Insurance Services

Tele. (561) 453-3395
Address: 601 S Federal Hwy, Suite 110, Boca Raton, FL 33432

Client Information Form

Please complete this form to ensure your prescriptions, doctors, and contact information are up to date for 2024. Please save the completed form and send it to us via email at service@acbs-llc.com Alternatively, you can mail it to the above address.

Name _____ **Date of Birth** _____

Address _____

Mailing Address (if Different) _____

Email _____ **Home:** _____ **Cell:** _____

Insurance & Physician's Information

Medicare Number _____ **MEDICAID** No

Medicare Effective Dates: Part A _____ **Part B** _____

Present Coverage _____

Are you satisfied with your current insurance policy? _____

PRIMARY CARE DOCTOR

_____

_____

SPECIALIST
_____

SPECIALIST
_____

SPECIALIST
_____

SPECIALIST
_____

SPECIALIST
_____

Preferred Hospital [ ]   Preferred Pharmacy [ ]

Medication Information

MEDICATION	DOSAGE |ex 20MG|	QTY & FREQUENCY

NOTES

NOTES

NOTES

NOTES

ABOUT THE AUTHOR

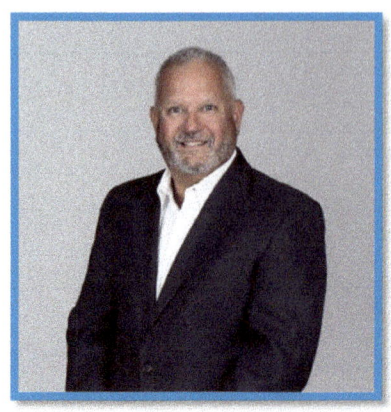

Lawrence Adkins is the CEO of ACBS, LLC, a Medicare and health insurance agency with multiple locations. Since taking the helm in May 2023, Lawrence has led the acquisition of several agencies, driving the company's growth. Previously, Lawrence was the Director of Mergers and Acquisitions at Smart Choice Partners LLC, where he played a key role in building the company from the ground up, completing 25 acquisitions in three years and contributing $6.2 million in revenue. Before that, he founded Ample Insurance LLC, expanding it to six locations and over $5.6 million in revenue through 23 acquisitions.

Lawrence Adkins began at Mutual of New York as a Financial Services Representative, where he quickly rose to become the top Financial Advisor. He has held leadership roles at MetLife as Regional Vice President, AXA as the President of the North America Division and has extensive experience managing teams and driving significant revenue growth, while keeping the customer at the heart of everything he does. Larry holds various insurance and financial licenses, as well as a Chartered Financial Consultant designation. Outside of work, he enjoys golf, exercise, fishing, and traveling. A devoted father of two daughters, he believes in supporting philanthropy and a portion of the proceeds of this book will support the ongoing programs of health and wellness, research, and funding for the Alzheimer's Foundation. For more information or to hire Lawrence Adkins to keynote at your next corporate function with a book signing please contact:

ladkins@acbs-llc.com

Retire with Peace of Mind

At ACBS Insurance Services, we are a nationally recognized independent insurance agency dedicated to providing unbiased assistance and support to seniors and their families in selecting Medicare insurance plan options that best suits their needs and budget. Our mission is to bring peace of mind to those entering retirement by simplifying the complex and often confusing process of securing quality, affordable healthcare. We understand that the array of healthcare options available through Medicare can be overwhelming, and the importance of adhering to specific timeframes and enrollment windows to retain crucial benefits cannot be overstated.

Seeing a gap in the insurance industry, ACBS Insurance Services was founded to offer a higher standard of service. As an independent agency representing a wide range of Medicare insurance plan options across the United States, we provide impartial guidance to help our clients choose the most appropriate coverage tailored to their unique situations. Through education, professional qualifications, and market analysis, we ensure our clients are well-informed and confident in their healthcare decisions. Our independence means our loyalty lies solely with our clients, not any insurance company. Our goal is to empower individuals with the knowledge they need to make the best healthcare choices.

We serve as a dedicated point of contact and advocate, guiding our clients through every step of the enrollment process and continually reassessing their coverage to adapt to changing needs, ensuring they always have the best possible insurance fit.

This book supports the ongoing efforts of the Alzheimer's Foundation 501.(C).3 with a portion of the book sales funding programs and research.

CEO of ACBS, LLC

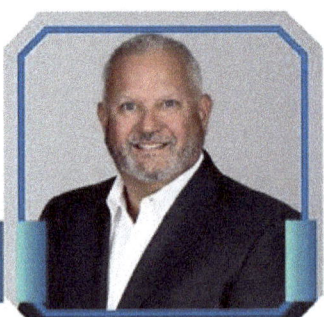

AUTHOR: LAWRENCE ADKINS

www.ingramcontent.com/pod-product-compliance
Lightning Source LLC
Chambersburg PA
CBHW062126040426
42337CB00044B/4326